WEIGHT GAIN
RECIPES COOKBOOK

*The Ultimate Guide to Gaining Weight the Right
Way through Healthy and Tasty Diet*

Bertha G. Baker

Table of Contents

INTRODUCTION 6

CHAPTER 1 8

Preparing for Weight Gain............................... 8

CHAPTER 2 12

Breakfast Recipes.. 12

1. Banana French Toast................................. 12

2. Oatmeal Pancakes 13

3. Egg and Avocado Toast.............................. 15

4. Peanut Butter and Banana Overnight Oats 16

5. Apple Cinnamon Oatmeal............................ 17

6. Bacon and Egg Breakfast Sandwich 18

7. Baked Oatmeal 20

8. Avocado Toast with Fried Egg 22

9. Omelette with Cheese and Spinach................... 23

10. Banana Protein Smoothie............................ 24

CHAPTER 3 26

Lunch Recipes.. 26

1. Fried Rice Bowl 26

2. Chili Cheese Fries 27

3. Chicken Parmesan................................... 29

4. Lasagna 31

5. Baked Macaroni and Cheese.. 33

6. Stuffed Peppers 34

7. Pizza Quesadillas 36

8. Shepherd's Pie 38

9. Chicken Pot Pie... 39

10. Cheeseburger Casserole 41

CHAPTER 4 44

Dinner Recipes.. 44

1. Slow Cooker Beef Stroganoff.. 44

2. Chicken Parmesan.. 46

3. Cheesy Bacon Stuffed Mushrooms.................................... 48

4. Baked Mac and Cheese 49

5. Stuffed Bell Peppers 51

6. Baked Salmon 53

7. Baked Ziti... 54

8. Baked Chicken and Rice 56

9. Creamy Baked Potatoes 58

10. Apple Crisp 60

CHAPTER 5 62

Snack Recipes 62

1. Peanut Butter Oatmeal Balls.. 62

2. Chocolate Chip Banana Bread 63

3. Apple Cinnamon Oatmeal Cookies 64

4. Banana Smoothie 65

5. Peanut Butter and Jelly Protein Shake: 66

CHAPTER 6 68

Smoothies & Shakes 68

1. Banana Oatmeal Smoothie 68

2. Peanut Butter Protein Shake 69

3. Chocolate Coconut Shake: 69

4. Strawberry Banana Smoothie 70

5. Avocado Mango Smoothie: 70

CHAPTER 7 72

Supplementation and Supplements 72

CONCLUSION 74

INTRODUCTION

Ashley had been struggling with her weight for some time now. Nothing appeared to work despite her attempts at every diet and workout plan she could discover. She had heard about some new weight-gain recipes and decided to give them a try.

At first, Ashley was skeptical. She had always been told that eating too much would make her gain weight. But the recipes she read about seemed healthy and balanced, so she decided to give it a try.

To her surprise, Ashley started gaining weight after only a few weeks of following the recipes. She was amazed at how quickly her body responded to the change in diet. She started to feel more energetic and her clothes fit better too.

Even though Ashley had gained some weight, she was thrilled with the results. She was eating healthier than ever before and still managing to put on some extra pounds.

As time went on, Ashley kept up with her new diet. She was careful to stick to the recipes and make sure she was getting all the necessary nutrients for her body to stay healthy.

After months of dedicated effort, Ashley had achieved her goal. She had gained the weight she desired and was feeling great. She was happy that she had found a way to gain weight in a healthy and balanced way.

Ashley was glad she had taken the plunge and tried something new. She was now more confident in her body than ever and was looking forward to maintaining her weight-gain success.

Welcome to our weight gain recipes book! Whether you're looking to put on some much-needed pounds or just want to add some extra muscle, we've got the recipes you need to make it happen.

Weight gain can be a necessity for a variety of reasons, including health, sports performance, or simply wanting to look good. Eating the right foods and increasing your calorie intake can be a great way to reach your goals.

In this book, you'll find delicious recipes that are easy to make and pack in the calories. With our recipes, you'll be able to gain weight while still eating healthy, balanced meals.

Weight gain is also important for people with certain medical conditions, such as those with a chronic illness or anorexia. In these cases, gaining weight can be essential for restoring health. Our recipes are tailored to meet the needs of these individuals, providing the nutrients and calories required for optimal health.

So, if you're looking for the perfect way to gain weight in a healthy way, you've come to the right place. Now, let's get cooking!

CHAPTER 1

Preparing for Weight Gain

Gaining weight is a common goal for many people. Whether it's to gain muscle mass, become healthier, or just to look better, gaining weight is something that many individuals strive for. However, it can be difficult to reach this goal without proper preparation. In this article, we will discuss 10 ways to prepare for weight gain.

1. Start Strength Training: Strength training is the best way to build muscle mass and gain weight. It is important to focus on compound exercises such as squats, deadlifts, bench press, overhead press, and rows. These exercises will help you build muscle mass more effectively than isolation exercises.

2. Increase Caloric Intake: In order to gain weight, you need to consume more calories than you burn. This means that you need to increase your caloric intake in order to gain weight. This can be done by adding healthy snacks between meals, or by increasing the portion sizes of your meals.

3. Eat Quality Foods: Eating quality foods is essential for gaining weight. You should focus on eating nutrient-dense foods such as lean proteins, complex carbohydrates, fruits, vegetables, and healthy fats. These foods will provide your body with the necessary nutrients it needs to build muscle and gain weight.

4. Drink Plenty of Water: It is important to stay hydrated when trying to gain weight. Drinking plenty of water will help you stay hydrated and help your body absorb nutrients more effectively.

5. Get Enough Sleep: Getting enough sleep is essential for gaining weight. When you sleep, your body releases growth hormone, which helps to build muscle and promote weight gain.

6. Take Supplements: Taking supplements can help you reach your weight gain goals faster. Supplements such as whey protein, creatine, and BCAAs can help you build muscle and gain weight more effectively.

7. Monitor Progress: Monitoring your progress is essential for gaining weight. You should weigh yourself and measure your body fat regularly so that you can track your progress and make adjustments as needed.

8. Be Consistent: Gaining weight takes time and dedication. You need to be consistent with your diet, exercise routine, and supplement intake in order to reach your weight gain goals.

9. Avoid Unhealthy Habits: Unhealthy habits such as smoking, drinking alcohol, and lack of sleep can have a negative effect on your weight gain goals. Avoiding these habits will help you reach your goals faster.

10. Stay Motivated: Gaining weight can be a long and difficult process. It is important to stay motivated and focus on your goals so that you can reach them.

Gaining weight can be a difficult and time-consuming process. However, with the right preparation and dedication, it is possible to reach your weight gain goals. These 10 tips can help you prepare for weight gain and reach your goals faster.

CHAPTER 2

Breakfast Recipes

1. Banana French Toast

Start off your day with a delicious and nutritious breakfast that is sure to provide you with the energy and calories to last throughout the day. This Banana French Toast is sure to do the trick!

Ingredients

- 2 slices of thick-cut brioche bread

- 2 eggs

- 1/2 cup of milk

- 1 banana, mashed

- 2 tablespoons of butter

- 1 teaspoon of cinnamon

- Pinch of nutmeg

- Maple syrup

Instructions:

1. Beat the eggs and milk together in a shallow bowl.

2. Dip the brioche slices into the egg mixture, turning to coat both sides.

3. In a separate bowl, mash the banana and add the cinnamon and nutmeg.

4. Spread the banana mixture onto one side of each slice of brioche.

5. Heat the butter in a large skillet over medium heat.

6. Place the brioche slices in the skillet, banana side down.

7. Cook for about 2 minutes, then carefully flip and cook for another 2 minutes.

8. Serve with maple syrup and enjoy!

2. Oatmeal Pancakes

Give your morning pancakes a nutritious makeover with these Oatmeal Pancakes. They are sure to provide you with the energy and calories your body needs to stay energized throughout the day.

Ingredients:

- 1 cup of rolled oats

- 2 eggs

- 1 cup of milk

- 2 tablespoons of honey

- 2 tablespoons of olive oil

- 2 tablespoons of baking powder

- Pinch of salt

Instructions:

1. In a large bowl, mix together the oats, eggs, milk, honey, olive oil, baking powder, and salt.

2. Heat a large skillet over medium heat.

3. Grease the skillet with butter or oil.

4. Pour 1/4 cup of the batter into the skillet and cook for 2-3 minutes per side.

5. Repeat with the remaining batter.

6. Serve with your favorite toppings and enjoy!

3. Egg and Avocado Toast

This Egg and Avocado Toast is the perfect way to start your day! It's packed with healthy fats and protein that will help you stay full and energized throughout the day.

Ingredients:

- 2 slices of whole wheat bread

- 2 eggs

- 1 avocado, mashed

- 2 tablespoons of olive oil

- Salt and pepper to taste

Instructions:

1. In a big skillet over medium heat, warm the olive oil.

2. Once the whites are set, add the cracked eggs to the skillet and cook for about 2 minutes.

3. In the meantime, toast the bread in the oven or with a toaster.

4. Cover the toast with the mashed avocado.

5. Place the eggs on top of the avocado and sprinkle with salt and pepper.

6. Enjoy your Egg and Avocado Toast!

4. Peanut Butter and Banana Overnight Oats

This Peanut Butter and Banana Overnight Oats recipe is the perfect grab-and-go breakfast to fuel your morning. It's packed with protein and healthy fats to help you stay full and energized throughout the day.

Ingredients:

- 1/2 cup of rolled oats

- 1/2 cup of mil

- 1 tablespoon of chia seeds

- 2 tablespoons of peanut butter

- 1 banana, sliced

Instructions:

1. In a medium bowl, mix together the oats, milk, and chia seeds.

2. Stir in the peanut butter until fully incorporated.

3. Add the sliced banana and mix well.

4. Cover the bowl and refrigerate overnight.

5. In the morning, take the bowl out of the refrigerator and enjoy!

5. Apple Cinnamon Oatmeal

This Apple Cinnamon Oatmeal is the perfect way to start your day. It's packed with fiber and protein to help you stay full and energized throughout the day.

Ingredients:

- 1 cup of rolled oat

- 2 cups of water

- 1 apple, diced

- 2 tablespoons of honey

- 2 teaspoons of cinnamon

- Pinch of salt

Instructions:

1. Bring the water to a boil in a medium saucepan.

2. Add the oats and turn the heat down to low.

3. Simmer for five minutes, stirring now and then.

4. Include the apple dice, honey, cinnamon, and salt.

5. Continue to simmer for an additional 5 minutes while stirring now and again.

6. Plate and enjoy with your favorite toppings!

6. Bacon and Egg Breakfast Sandwich

This Bacon and Egg Breakfast Sandwich is a delicious and easy way to start your day. It's packed with protein and healthy fats to help you stay full and energized throughout the day.

Ingredients:

- 2 slices of whole wheat bread

- 2 eggs

- 2 slices of bacon

- 2 slices of cheese

- 2 tablespoons of butter

Instructions:

1. Heat a large skillet over medium heat.

2. Add the bacon and cook for about 5 minutes, or until crispy.

3. Meanwhile, in a separate bowl, beat the eggs.

4. Add the eggs to the skillet and scramble until cooked through.

5. Spread the butter on one side of each slice of bread.

6. Place the slices of bread in the skillet, butter side down.

7. Top one slice of bread with the bacon, eggs, and cheese.

8. Place the other slice of bread on top, butter side up.

9. Cook for about 2 minutes, or until the cheese is melted and the bread is golden brown.

10. Serve and enjoy!

7. Baked Oatmeal

This Baked Oatmeal is a delicious and nutritious way to start your day. It's packed with fiber and protein to help you stay full and energized throughout the day.

Ingredients:

- 2 cups of rolled oats

- 1 teaspoon of baking powder

- 1 teaspoon of cinnamon

- 1/4 teaspoon of salt

- 2 eggs

- 1 cup of milk

- 1/4 cup of melted butter

- 1/2 cup of brown sugar

- 1 teaspoon of vanilla extract

- 1 cup of blueberries

Instructions:

1. Preheat the oven to 350°F.

2. In a large bowl, mix together the oats, baking powder, cinnamon, and salt.

3. In a separate bowl, whisk together the eggs, milk, melted butter, brown sugar, and vanilla extract.

4. Add the wet ingredients to the dry ingredients and mix until combined.

5. Fold in the blueberries.

6. Grease an 8x8-inch baking dish and pour the oatmeal mixture in.

7. Bake for 35-40 minutes, or until golden brown.

8. Serve warm and enjoy!

8. Avocado Toast with Fried Egg

This Avocado Toast with Fried Egg is an easy and delicious way to start your day. It's packed with healthy fats and protein to help you stay full and energized throughout the day.

Ingredients:

- 2 slices of whole wheat bread

- 1 avocado, mashed

- 2 eggs

- 2 tablespoons of olive oil

- Salt and pepper to taste

Instructions:

1. Use a toaster or the oven to toast the bread.

2. Cover the toast with the mashed avocado.

3. In a big skillet over medium heat, warm the olive oil.

4. Crack the eggs into the skillet and cook for about 2 minutes, or until the whites are set.

5. Place the eggs on top of the avocado and sprinkle with salt and pepper.

6. Serve and enjoy!

9. Omelette with Cheese and Spinach

This Omelette with Cheese and Spinach is a delicious and nutritious way to start your day. It's packed with protein and healthy fats to help you stay full and energized throughout the day.

Ingredients:

- 2 eggs

- 2 tablespoons of milk

- 2 tablespoons of butter

- 1/4 cup of grated cheese

- 1/4 cup of chopped spinach

- Salt and pepper to taste

Instructions:

1. Whisk the eggs and milk together in a medium bowl.

2. Put a large skillet over medium heat and add the butter.

3. Add the egg mixture to the skillet and cook, stirring occasionally, until nearly set

4. Add the cheese and spinach and stir until the cheese is melted.

5. Fold the omelette in half and cook for an additional minute.

6. Slide the omelette onto a plate and season with salt and pepper.

7. Serve and enjoy!

10. Banana Protein Smoothie

This Banana Protein Smoothie is the perfect grab-and-go breakfast to fuel your morning. It's packed with protein and healthy fats to help you stay full and energized throughout the day.

Ingredients:

- 1 banana, sliced

- 1/2 cup of plain Greek yogurt

- 1/2 cup of almond milk

- 1/4 cup of rolled oats

- 2 tablespoons of peanut butter

- 1 tablespoon of honey

- Pinch of cinnamon

Instructions:

1. In a blender, combine all the ingredients and process until completely smooth.

2. Transfer the smoothie to a glass, then sip it.

3. You can also pour the smoothie into a resealable container and store in the refrigerator for up to 2 days.

CHAPTER 3

Lunch Recipes

1. Fried Rice Bowl

This Fried Rice Bowl is a delicious and hearty lunch that will leave you feeling satisfied and energized. It is packed full of flavor and nutrients from all of the vegetables, and the addition of fried rice makes it a great way to get your daily dose of carbs.

Ingredients:

- 2 cups cooked white or brown rice

- 2 tablespoons sesame oil

- 1 small onion, diced

- 2 cloves garlic, minced

- 2 carrots, diced

- 1 bell pepper, diced

- 2 cups chopped broccoli

- 2 tablespoons soy sauce

- 2 teaspoons sugar

- Salt and pepper to taste

Instructions:

1. Heat sesame oil in a large skillet over medium heat.

2. Add onion and garlic and cook until softened, about 5 minutes.

3. Add carrots, bell pepper and broccoli and cook until tender, about 8 minutes.

4. Add cooked rice to the pan and cook until heated through, about 5 minutes.

5. Mix in soy sauce, sugar, salt and pepper.

6. Serve warm.

2. Chili Cheese Fries

Chili Cheese Fries are a classic comfort food that is sure to satisfy your cravings. This dish is packed with protein and carbs, making it an ideal lunch for weight gain.

Ingredients:

- 2 potatoes, cut into wedges

- 2 tablespoons olive oil

- Salt and pepper to taste

- 2 cups cooked ground beef

- 1 can (14.5 oz) diced tomatoes

- 1 can (15 oz) black beans, rinsed and drained

- 1 teaspoon chili powder

- 2 cups shredded cheddar cheese

- 2 tablespoons chopped fresh cilantro

Instructions:

1. Preheat oven to 400°F.

2. Place potato wedges on a baking sheet and drizzle with olive oil. Sprinkle with salt and pepper.

3. Bake for 20 minutes, flipping halfway through.

4. Meanwhile, in a large skillet, cook ground beef over medium heat until no longer pink.

5. Add tomatoes, beans, chili powder and a pinch of salt and pepper. Simmer for 10 minutes.

6. Place cooked potato wedges on a serving dish and top with chili mixture and cheese.

7. Bake for 10 minutes or until cheese is melted.

8. Garnish with cilantro before serving.

3. Chicken Parmesan

Chicken Parmesan is a classic Italian dish that is sure to please. This version is loaded with cheese and carbs, making it a great choice for those looking to gain weight.

Ingredients:

- 2 boneless, skinless chicken breasts

- 1 cup Italian-style breadcrumbs

- 1/2 cup grated Parmesan cheese

- 1 teaspoon Italian seasoning

- Salt and pepper to taste

- 2 eggs

- 2 tablespoons olive oil

- 1/2 cup marinara sauce

- 1/2 cup shredded mozzarella cheese

Instructions:

1. Preheat oven to 350°F.

2. In a shallow bowl, mix together breadcrumbs, Parmesan cheese, Italian seasoning and a pinch of salt and pepper.

3. In a separate bowl, beat eggs.

4. Dip chicken into egg mixture, then coat with breadcrumb mixture.

5. Heat olive oil in a large skillet over medium heat.

6. Add chicken to skillet and cook for 5 minutes on each side.

7. Transfer chicken to a baking dish and top with marinara sauce and mozzarella cheese.

8. Bake for 15 minutes or until chicken is cooked through.

4. Lasagna

Lasagna is a classic Italian dish that is sure to please. This version is loaded with cheese and carbs, making it a great choice for those looking to gain weight.

Ingredients:

- 1 pound ground beef

- 1/2 onion, diced

- 2 cloves garlic, minced

- 1 can (28 oz) diced tomatoes

- 1 can (6 oz) tomato paste

- 1 teaspoon Italian seasoning

- Salt and pepper to taste

- 9 lasagna noodles

- 2 cups ricotta cheese

- 1/2 cup grated Parmesan cheese

- 2 cups shredded mozzarella cheese

Instructions:

1. Preheat oven to 375°F.

2. In a large skillet, cook ground beef, onion, and garlic over medium heat until no longer pink.

3. Add tomatoes, tomato paste, Italian seasoning and a pinch of salt and pepper. Simmer for 10 minutes.

4. Spread 1 cup of meat sauce in the bottom of a 9x13 inch baking dish.

5. Place 3 lasagna noodles on top, then spread with 1/2 of the ricotta cheese and 1/2 of the Parmesan cheese.

6. Top with 1/2 of the meat sauce and 1/2 of the mozzarella cheese.

7. Repeat layers, ending with mozzarella cheese on top.

8. Cover with foil and bake for 25 minutes.

9. Remove foil and bake for an additional 10 minutes.

10. Let lasagna rest for 10 minutes before serving.

5. Baked Macaroni and Cheese

Baked Macaroni and Cheese is a classic comfort food that is sure to satisfy your cravings. This version is loaded with cheese and carbs, making it a great choice for those looking to gain weight.

Ingredients:

- 2 cups uncooked elbow macaroni

- 2 tablespoons butter

- 2 tablespoons all-purpose flour

- 2 cups milk

- 2 cups shredded cheddar cheese

- 1/2 teaspoon dry mustard

- Salt and pepper to taste

- 1/2 cup grated Parmesan cheese

Instructions:

1. Preheat oven to 375°F.

2. Cook macaroni according to package instructions.

3. Meanwhile, melt butter in a large saucepan over medium heat.

4. Add flour and whisk until combined.

5. Slowly add milk, whisking constantly until sauce is thick and bubbly.

6. Add cheddar cheese and dry mustard and stir until cheese is melted.

7. Add salt and pepper to taste.

8. Drain macaroni and add to sauce, stirring to combine.

9. Transfer macaroni to a greased 9x13 inch baking dish and sprinkle with Parmesan cheese.

10. Bake for 20 minutes or until cheese is golden and bubbly.

6. Stuffed Peppers

Stuffed peppers are a great way to get a healthy dose of vegetables and protein. This version is also loaded with carbs, making it a great choice for those looking to gain weight.

Ingredients:

- 4 bell peppers, halved and seeded

- 1 pound ground beef

- 1 onion, diced

- 2 cloves garlic, minced

- 1 can (14.5 oz) diced tomatoes

- 1 cup uncooked white rice

- 1 teaspoon Italian seasoning

- Salt and pepper to taste

- 1 cup shredded mozzarella cheese

Instructions:

1. Preheat oven to 375°F.

2. Place bell pepper halves in a greased 9x13 inch baking dish.

3. In a large skillet, cook ground beef, onion and garlic over medium heat until no longer pink.

4. Add tomatoes, rice, Italian seasoning and a pinch of salt and pepper. Simmer for 10 minutes.

5. Fill bell pepper halves with beef mixture.

6. Top with mozzarella cheese.

7. Bake for 20 minutes or until cheese is melted and bubbly.

7. Pizza Quesadillas

Pizza Quesadillas are a delicious and easy way to get your pizza fix. These quesadillas are packed with cheese and carbs, making them a great choice for those looking to gain weight.

Ingredients:

- 4 large flour tortillas

- 2 cups shredded mozzarella cheese

- 1/2 cup pizza sauce

- 1/2 cup sliced pepperoni

- 2 tablespoons butter, melted

Instructions:

1. Preheat a large skillet over medium heat.

2. Place one tortilla in the skillet.

3. Sprinkle with 1/2 cup of the mozzarella cheese and top with pepperoni.

4. Spread 1/4 cup of pizza sauce over the pepperoni.

5. Top with another tortilla and press down lightly.

6. Brush top with melted butter.

7. Flip over and cook for 3 minutes or until golden brown.

8. Flip quesadilla over and cook for an additional 3 minutes.

9. Remove from skillet and repeat with remaining ingredients.

10. Cut into wedges and serve.

8. Shepherd's Pie

Shepherd's Pie is a classic comfort food that is sure to satisfy your cravings. This version is packed with protein and carbs, making it an ideal lunch for weight gain.

Ingredients:

- 2 tablespoons olive oil

- 1 onion, diced

- 2 cloves garlic, minced

- 1 pound ground beef

- 1 can (14.5 oz) diced tomatoes

- 1 teaspoon Italian seasoning

- Salt and pepper to taste

- 3 cups mashed potatoes

- 1 cup shredded cheddar cheese

Instructions:

1. Preheat oven to 375°F.

2. Heat olive oil in a large skillet over medium heat.

3. Add onion and garlic and cook until softened, about 5 minutes.

4. Add ground beef and cook until no longer pink.

5. Add tomatoes, Italian seasoning and a pinch of salt and pepper. Simmer for 10 minutes.

6. Spread beef mixture in the bottom of a 9x13 inch baking dish.

7. Spread mashed potatoes over the top and sprinkle with cheddar cheese.

8. Bake for 25 minutes or until cheese is melted and bubbly.

9. Let sit for 10 minutes before serving.

9. Chicken Pot Pie

Chicken Pot Pie is a classic comfort food that is sure to satisfy your cravings. This version is packed with protein and carbs, making it an ideal lunch for weight gain.

Ingredients:

- 2 tablespoons butter

- 1 onion, diced

- 2 carrots, diced

- 2 stalks celery, diced

- 2 cloves garlic, minced

- 2 tablespoons all-purpose flour

- 2 cups chicken broth

- 2 cups cooked, shredded chicken

- 1 cup frozen peas

- 1/2 cup heavy cream

- Salt and pepper to taste

- 2 pie crusts

Instructions:

1. Preheat oven to 375°F.

2. Heat butter in a large skillet over medium heat.

3. Add onion, carrots, celery and garlic and cook until softened, about 8 minutes.

4. Stir in flour and cook for 1 minute.

5. Slowly add chicken broth, stirring constantly, until mixture is thick and bubbly.

6. Add chicken, peas, cream and a pinch of salt and pepper. Simmer for 10 minutes.

7. Pour chicken mixture into a 9-inch pie dish.

8. Place one pie crust on top and press down lightly.

9. Cut several slits in the top of the crust to allow steam to escape.

10. Bake for 30 minutes or until crust is golden brown.

10. Cheeseburger Casserole

Cheeseburger Casserole is a delicious and hearty dish that is sure to satisfy your cravings. This version is packed with protein and carbs, making it an ideal lunch for weight gain.

Ingredients:

- 1 pound ground beef

- 1 onion, diced

- 2 cloves garlic, minced

- 1 teaspoon Worcestershire sauce

- 1 teaspoon Italian seasoning

- Salt and pepper to taste

- 4 cups cooked macaroni

- 1 can (10.5 oz) cream of mushroom soup

- 2 cups shredded cheddar cheese

Instructions:

1. Preheat oven to 375°F.

2. In a large skillet, cook ground beef, onion and garlic over medium heat until no longer pink.

3. Add Worcestershire sauce, Italian seasoning and a pinch of salt and pepper. Simmer for 10 minutes.

4. In a large bowl, combine cooked macaroni, soup and 1 cup of the cheddar cheese.

5. Add ground beef mixture and stir to combine.

6. Transfer mixture to a greased 9x13 inch baking dish and top with remaining 1 cup of cheddar cheese.

7. Bake for 25 minutes or until cheese is melted and bubbly.

8. Let casserole rest for 10 minutes before serving.

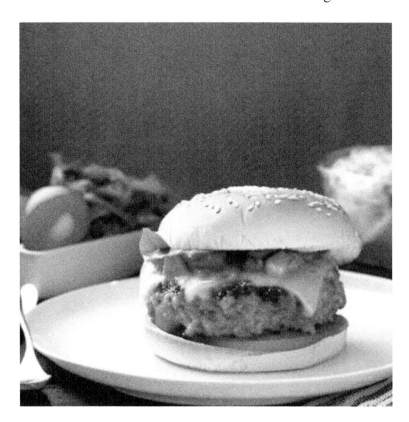

CHAPTER 4

Dinner Recipes

1. Slow Cooker Beef Stroganoff

This classic beef stroganoff is made easier with the help of a slow cooker. The tender beef, mushrooms, and onions are cooked in a rich and creamy sauce that is full of flavor.

Ingredients:

- 2 pounds beef stew meat

- 2 tablespoons olive oil

- 1 onion, chopped

- 8 ounces mushrooms, sliced

- 2 cloves garlic, minced

- 2 tablespoons all-purpose flour

- 2 teaspoons paprika

- 1 teaspoon salt

- 1/4 teaspoon pepper

- 2 cups beef broth

- 2 tablespoons Worcestershire sauce

- 1/2 cup sour cream

Instructions:

1. In a big skillet, heat the olive oil over medium-high heat.

2. Include the beef, and cook it for 5-7 minutes, or until it is browned.

3. Transfer the beef to the slow cooker and add the onion, mushrooms, and garlic to the skillet.

4. Cook for 5 minutes, or until the vegetables are tender.

5. Add the flour, paprika, salt, and pepper to the skillet and stir to combine.

6. Slowly pour in the beef broth and Worcestershire sauce and stir until the mixture is smooth.

7. Pour the mixture over the beef and vegetables in the slow cooker.

8. Cover and cook on low for 6-8 hours, or until the beef is tender.

9. Stir in the sour cream and season with additional salt and pepper, if desired.

10. Serve over cooked egg noodles or mashed potatoes.

2. Chicken Parmesan

The entire family will enjoy this traditional Italian dish.

The chicken is breaded and fried, then topped with a flavorful marinara sauce and melted cheese.

Ingredients:

- 4 boneless skinless chicken breasts

- 1/2 cup all-purpose flour

- 2 eggs, beaten

- 2 cups Italian-style bread crumbs

- 1/4 cup olive oil

- 2 cups marinara sauce

- 1/2 cup grated Parmesan cheese

- 1/2 cup shredded mozzarella cheese

Instructions:

1. Set the oven's temperature to 350 degrees Fahrenheit.

2. Put the flour in a small bowl.

3. Put the eggs in a another shallow bowl.

4. Put the bread crumbs in a third shallow basin.

5. Dredge each chicken breast in flour, then in eggs, and last in bread crumbs.

6. In a large skillet over medium-high heat, warm the olive oil.

7. Add the chicken and cook for 4-5 minutes per side, or until golden brown and cooked through.

8. Transfer the chicken to a baking dish.

9. Top with the marinara sauce and sprinkle with the Parmesan and mozzarella cheese.

10. Bake for 15 minutes, or until the cheese is melted and bubbly.

3. Cheesy Bacon Stuffed Mushrooms

These cheesy bacon stuffed mushrooms are a delicious appetizer or side dish. The mushrooms are filled with a mixture of bacon, cream cheese, and Parmesan cheese and baked until golden and bubbly.

Ingredients:

- 24 large mushrooms

- 6 slices bacon, cooked and crumbled

- 8 ounces cream cheese, softened

- 1/4 cup grated Parmesan cheese

- 1/4 teaspoon garlic powder

- 1/4 teaspoon onion powder

- Salt and pepper, to taste

- 2 tablespoons chopped fresh parsley

Instructions: 1. Set the oven's temperature to 350 degrees Fahrenheit.

2. Remove the stems from the mushrooms and set aside.

3. In a medium bowl, combine the bacon, cream cheese, Parmesan cheese, garlic powder, onion powder, salt, and pepper.

4. Spoon the mixture into the mushroom caps.

5. Place the mushrooms on a baking sheet and bake for 15-20 minutes, or until golden and bubbly.

6. Sprinkle with the parsley and serve.

4. Baked Mac and Cheese

This traditional baked mac and cheese is rich, cheesy, and scrumptious! The macaroni is baked in a creamy cheese sauce and topped with crunchy bread crumbs for the perfect comfort food.

Ingredients:

- 1 pound elbow macaroni

- 2 tablespoons butter

- 2 tablespoons all-purpose flour

- 2 cups milk

- 2 cups shredded cheddar cheese

- 1/2 cup grated Parmesan cheese

- 1/4 teaspoon salt

- 1/4 teaspoon pepper

- 1/4 teaspoon garlic powder

- 1/4 cup bread crumbs

Instructions:

1. Set the oven's temperature to 350 F.

2. Cook the macaroni as directed on the packet.

3. Set the macaroni aside after draining.

4. In a big pot over medium heat, melt the butter. \

5. Include the flour and mix to combine.

6. Stir continuously as you gradually add the milk until the liquid is thick and bubbling.

7. Turn off the heat and add the cheddar and Parmesan cheeses, together with the salt, pepper, and garlic powder.]

8. Combine the cheese sauce and cooked macaroni by adding both to a bowl.

9. Place the mixture in a baking dish that has been buttered.

10. Top with bread crumbs and bake for 25 to 30 minutes, or until bubbling and golden.

5. Stuffed Bell Peppers

These stuffed bell peppers are full of flavor and nutrition. The bell peppers are stuffed with a mixture of ground beef, rice, tomatoes, and cheese and baked until tender.

Ingredients:

- 4 large bell peppers

- 1 pound ground beef

- 1 onion, chopped

- 1 cup cooked rice

- 1 can (14.5 ounces) diced tomatoes

- 1 teaspoon garlic powder

- 1/2 teaspoon salt

- 1/4 teaspoon pepper

- 1 cup shredded cheddar cheese

Instructions:

1. Preheat the oven to 350 degrees F.

2. Cut the tops off the bell peppers and remove the seeds and membranes.

3. Place the bell peppers in a baking dish.

4. In a large skillet over medium-high heat, cook the ground beef and onion until the beef is no longer pink.

5. Drain off any excess fat.

6. Add the rice, tomatoes, garlic powder, salt, and pepper and stir to combine.

7. Spoon the mixture into the bell peppers.

8. Top with the cheddar cheese.

9. Cover the baking dish with aluminum foil.

10. Bake for 45 minutes, or until the peppers are tender.

6. Baked Salmon

This easy baked salmon is a delicious and healthy meal. The fish is seasoned with a lemon garlic butter sauce and baked until it is flaky and tender.

Ingredients:

- 4 salmon fillets

- 2 tablespoons butter, melted

- 2 cloves garlic, minced

- 2 tablespoons lemon juice

- 1 teaspoon dried parsley

- 1/2 teaspoon salt

- 1/4 teaspoon pepper

Instructions:

1. Preheat the oven to 400 degrees F.

2. Place the salmon fillets on a greased baking sheet.

3. In a small bowl, combine the butter, garlic, lemon juice, parsley, salt, and pepper.

4. Spread the butter mixture over the salmon.

5. Bake for 15-20 minutes, or until the salmon is cooked through.

6. Serve with a side of your favorite vegetables.

7. Baked Ziti

This baked ziti is a hearty and comforting dish. The ziti is cooked in a flavorful tomato sauce and topped with mozzarella and Parmesan cheese and baked until golden and bubbly.

Ingredients:

- 1 pound ziti

- 2 tablespoons olive oil

- 1 onion, chopped

- 2 cloves garlic, minced

- 2 cans (14.5 ounces each) diced tomatoes

- 1 teaspoon sugar

- 1 teaspoon dried oregano

- 1/2 teaspoon salt

- 1/4 teaspoon pepper

- 2 cups shredded mozzarella cheese

- 1/2 cup grated Parmesan cheese

Instructions:

1. Preheat the oven to 350 degrees F.

2. Cook the ziti according to the package directions.

3. Drain the ziti and set aside.

4. Heat the olive oil in a large skillet over medium heat.

5. Add the onion and garlic and cook for 5 minutes, or until softened.

6. Add the tomatoes, sugar, oregano, salt, and pepper and stir to combine.

7. Simmer for 10 minutes.

8. Add the cooked ziti to the skillet and stir to combine.

9. Transfer the mixture to a greased 9x13-inch baking dish.

10. Sprinkle with the mozzarella and Parmesan cheese.

11. Bake for 20 minutes, or until the cheese is melted and bubbly.

8. Baked Chicken and Rice

This baked chicken and rice is a one-pan meal that the whole family will love. The chicken is cooked in a flavorful tomato sauce with rice and topped with mozzarella cheese for a delicious and easy dinner.

Ingredients:

- 4 boneless skinless chicken breasts

- 2 tablespoons olive oil

- 1 onion, chopped

- 2 cloves garlic, minced

- 2 cans (14.5 ounces each) diced tomatoes

- 1 teaspoon sugar

- 1 teaspoon dried oregano

- 1/2 teaspoon salt

- 1/4 teaspoon pepper

- 1 cup uncooked white rice

- 2 cups chicken broth

- 1 cup shredded mozzarella cheese

Instructions:

1. Preheat the oven to 350 degrees F.

2. Heat the olive oil in a large skillet over medium heat.

3. Add the chicken and cook for 5 minutes per side, or until golden brown.

4. Remove the chicken from the skillet and set aside.

5. Add the onion and garlic to the skillet and cook for 5 minutes, or until softened.

6. Add the tomatoes, sugar, oregano, salt, and pepper and stir to combine.

7. Add the rice and chicken broth and stir to combine.

8. Place the chicken on top of the rice mixture.

9. Cover and bake for 45 minutes, or until the chicken is cooked through and the rice is tender.

10. Sprinkle with the mozzarella cheese and bake for an additional 10 minutes, or until the cheese is melted.

9. Creamy Baked Potatoes

These creamy baked potatoes are a delicious side dish. The potatoes are baked until tender and then filled with a creamy cheese sauce for the perfect comfort food.

Ingredients:

- 4 large potatoes

- 2 tablespoons butter

- 2 tablespoons all-purpose flour

- 2 cups milk

- 1 teaspoon garlic powder

- 1/4 teaspoon salt

- 1/4 teaspoon pepper

- 1/2 cup shredded cheddar cheese

- 1/4 cup grated Parmesan cheese

Instructions:

1. Preheat the oven to 400 degrees F.

2. Pierce the potatoes with a fork and place on a baking sheet.

3. Bake for 45 minutes, or until tender.

4. Cut the potatoes in half lengthwise and scoop out the insides, leaving a thin shell.

5. Mash the potato insides.

6. Melt the butter in a large saucepan over medium heat.

7. Add the flour and stir until smooth.

8. Gradually add the milk, stirring constantly, until the mixture is thick and bubbly.

9. Remove the pan from the heat and stir in the garlic powder, salt, pepper, cheddar cheese, and Parmesan cheese.

10. Spoon the cheese mixture into the potato shells and place on the baking sheet.

11. Bake for 15 minutes, or until golden and bubbly.

10. Apple Crisp

This apple crisp is a delicious and easy dessert. The apples are topped with a crunchy oat topping and baked until golden and bubbly.

Ingredients:

- 6 apples, peeled, cored, and sliced

- 2 tablespoons lemon juice

- 1/4 cup brown sugar

- 1/2 cup all-purpose flour

- 1/2 cup rolled oats

- 1/2 cup butter, melted

- 1/2 teaspoon ground cinnamon

- 1/4 teaspoon ground nutmeg

- 1/4 teaspoon salt

Instructions:

1. Preheat the oven to 350 degrees F.

2. Place the apples in a 9x13-inch baking dish and sprinkle with the lemon juice.

3. In a medium bowl, combine the brown sugar, flour, oats, butter, cinnamon, nutmeg, and salt and stir until crumbly.

4. Sprinkle the mixture over the apples.

5. Bake for 45 minutes, or until the apples are tender and the topping is golden and crisp.

6. Serve warm with a scoop of ice cream.

CHAPTER 5

Snack Recipes

1. Peanut Butter Oatmeal Balls

Ingredients:

-1/2 cup creamy peanut butter

-1/4 cup honey

-1/4 cup ground flaxseed

-1/4 cup old-fashioned rolled oats

-2 tablespoons mini chocolate chips

Instructions:

1. In a medium bowl, mix together the peanut butter, honey, and flaxseed until combined

2. Combine the oats and chocolate chips by stirring them together.

3. Roll the mixture into 1-inch balls and place on a parchment-lined baking sheet.

4. Before serving, place in the fridge for at least 30 minutes.

5. Enjoy!

2. Chocolate Chip Banana Bread

Ingredients:

-2 large ripe bananas, mashed

-1/3 cup melted butter

-1/2 cup light brown sugar

-1 teaspoon vanilla extract

-1 teaspoon baking powder

-1/2 teaspoon baking soda

-1/2 teaspoon salt

-1 and 1/2 cups all-purpose flour

-1/2 cup semi-sweet chocolate chips

Instructions:

1. Preheat oven to 350 degrees F. Cooking spray should be used to grease a 9x5-inch loaf pan.

2. In a medium bowl, mix together the mashed bananas, melted butter, brown sugar, and vanilla extract until combined.

3. In a separate bowl, whisk together the baking powder, baking soda, salt, and all-purpose flour.

4. Slowly add the dry ingredients to the wet ingredients, stirring until combined.

5. Fold in the chocolate chips.

6. Pour the batter into the prepared loaf pan and bake for 50-60 minutes, or until a toothpick inserted into the center comes out clean.

7. Let cool for 10 minutes before slicing and serving. Enjoy!

3. Apple Cinnamon Oatmeal Cookies

Ingredients:

-1/2 cup butter, softened

-1/2 cup light brown sugar

-1/4 cup granulated sugar

-1 egg

-1 teaspoon vanilla extract

-1 cup all-purpose flour

-1 teaspoon baking powder

-1/2 teaspoon baking soda

-1/2 teaspoon ground cinnamon

-1/4 teaspoon salt

-1 and 1/2 cups old-fashioned rolled oats

-1 large apple, peeled and diced

Instructions:

1. Preheat oven to 350 degrees F. Set aside two baking sheets that have been lined with parchment paper.

2. In a large bowl, cream together the butter and sugars until light and fluffy

3. Once mixed, add the egg and vanilla essence.

4. In a separate bowl, whisk together the flour, baking powder, baking soda, cinnamon, and salt.

5. Slowly add the dry ingredients to the wet ingredients, stirring until combined.

6. Stir in the oats and diced apple until combined.

7. Approximately 2 inches apart, drop tablespoonfuls of the dough onto the prepared baking sheets.

8. Bake for 12-14 minutes, or until the edges are golden brown.

9. Transfer to a wire rack to finish cooling entirely after cooling for 5 minutes on the baking sheets. Enjoy!

4. Banana Smoothie

Ingredients:

-1 large banana, frozen and cut into chunks

-1 cup plain Greek yogurt

-1/2 cup milk

-1 tablespoon honey

-1 teaspoon ground cinnamon

Instructions:

1. Place the banana, yogurt, milk, honey, and cinnamon in a blender.

2. Blend until smooth and creamy.

3. Pour into glasses and enjoy!

5. Peanut Butter and Jelly Protein Shake:

Ingredients:

-1/2 cup plain Greek yogurt

-1/2 cup milk

-2 tablespoons creamy peanut butter

-1/4 cup frozen berries

-1 scoop vanilla protein powder

Instructions:

1. Place the yogurt, milk, peanut butter, berries, and protein powder in a blender.

2. Blend until smooth and creamy.

3. Pour into glasses and enjoy!

CHAPTER 6

Smoothies & Shakes

1. Banana Oatmeal Smoothie

Ingredients:

-1 banana

-1/4 cup of uncooked oats

-1/2 cup of Greek yogurt

-1/4 cup of almond milk

-1 tablespoon of honey

-1/2 teaspoon of vanilla extract

Instructions:

In a blender, combine all ingredients and process until perfectly smooth. Serve chilled.

2. Peanut Butter Protein Shake

Ingredients:

-1 cup of almond milk

-1 scoop of vanilla protein powder

-2 tablespoons of peanut butter

-1 banana

-1/4 teaspoon of cinnamon

Instructions:

In a blender, combine all ingredients and process until perfectly smooth. Serve chilled.

3. Chocolate Coconut Shake:

Ingredients:

-1 cup of almond milk

-1 scoop of chocolate protein powder

-2 tablespoons of coconut flakes

-1 banana

-1 tablespoon of cocoa powder

Instructions:

In a blender, combine all ingredients and process until perfectly smooth. Serve chilled.

4. Strawberry Banana Smoothie

Ingredients:

-1 cup of almond milk

-1 scoop of vanilla protein powder

-1/2 cup of fresh or frozen strawberries

-1 banana

-1 tablespoon of honey

Instructions:

In a blender, combine all ingredients and process until perfectly smooth. Serve chilled.

5. Avocado Mango Smoothie:

Ingredients:

-1 cup of almond milk

-1 scoop of vanilla protein powder

-1/2 cup of diced mango

-1/4 of a ripe avocado

-1 tablespoon of honey

Instructions:

In a blender, combine all ingredients and process until perfectly smooth. Serve chilled.

CHAPTER 7

Supplementation and Supplements

Supplementation is the act of taking vitamins, minerals, and other nutrients in order to improve health and athletic performance. Many individuals use supplementation to fill in dietary gaps, improve overall health, and enhance physical performance.

When trying to gain weight, supplementation can be beneficial in providing the body with the extra nutrients needed to build muscle and gain weight. Here are seven supplements to consider when trying to gain weight:

1. Creatine: Creatine is a natural compound that helps to increase muscle growth, strength, and power

2. Protein Powder: Protein powder is a supplement made from whey, casein, or plant protein. It is often used to help build muscle mass and provide energy for workouts.

3. Weight Gainers: Weight gainers are supplements designed to help individuals gain weight. They typically contain high amounts of protein, carbohydrates, and fats.

4. Pre-Workout Supplements: Pre-workout supplements are designed to help boost energy and performance during workouts.

5. Glutamine: Glutamine is an amino acid that helps to promote muscle growth and recovery. Additionally, it can lessen soreness and fatigue following a workout session.

6. Vitamins and Minerals: Taking a multivitamin supplement can help to ensure that you are getting all the essential vitamins and minerals your body needs.

7. Omega-3 Fatty Acids: Omega-3 fatty acids are beneficial for promoting muscle growth and overall health. They could also help reduce inflammation. In addition to the supplements listed above, it is important to remember that proper nutrition and exercise are key components of any weight gain program For best results, supplements should be taken along with a healthy diet and frequent exercise.

CONCLUSION

Weight gain is a frequent problem that some people struggle with. Having a healthy diet and regular exercise is the best way to gain weight in a healthy, sustainable way. This book of weight gain recipes provides delicious and nutritious recipes that can help you reach your health and fitness goals.

The recipes in this book are designed to be easy to make, tasty, and provide your body with the energy and nutrients it needs to gain weight. All of the recipes include healthy proteins, healthy fats, complex carbohydrates, fruits and vegetables, and other nutrient-dense ingredients. The recipes are also low in added sugar and sodium, and many of them are vegan-friendly.

Overall, this book of weight gain recipes offers a great way for those who are looking to gain weight in a healthy way. All of the recipes are delicious and nutritious, and provide your body with the energy and nutrients it needs to reach your weight gain goals. With regular exercise and a balanced diet, you can start to see results in no time.

Printed in Great Britain
by Amazon

44417834R00044